31 Days of Down Syndrome:

A Handbook for Special Families

by

Cheryl Patterson, Author
Ray Patterson, Co-Author

DORRANCE
PUBLISHING CO
EST. 1920
PITTSBURGH, PENNSYLVANIA 15238

The contents of this work, including, but not limited to, the accuracy of events, people, and places depicted; opinions expressed; permission to use previously published materials included; and any advice given or actions advocated are solely the responsibility of the author, who assumes all liability for said work and indemnifies the publisher against any claims stemming from publication of the work.

Dorrance Publishing Co
585 Alpha Drive
Pittsburgh, PA 15238
Visit our website at *www.dorrancebookstore.com*

ISBN: 978-1-6491-3420-2
eISBN: 978-1-6491-3552-0

Contents

A Short Story

Once upon a time…a King, his Queen, and their Princess lived beyond happily in a kingdom of peace and joy until one day their lives were unexpectedly changed when the King was mysteriously greeted by a short, darkly cloaked individual who reached out to the King and began to speak.

"Are you a good person?" asked the cloaked individual. The King seemed shocked, as this was no one he had ever met in his kingdom before. You see… the King was proud of his family, proud of his people, and proud to know he knew everyone in his kingdom.

Taking a deep breath, while puffing up his chest, the King exclaimed, "I am a good father, a good husband, and a good King." The cloaked person offered the King a basket, but the King could only see that in the basket was what seemed to be a rolled blanket.

The cloaked person then said to the King, "Take this…it is yours for now. When I return, if you have not proven to be a changed person, you will lose all you have." The King quickly turned to the Queen, stunned that a stranger would suggest such a thing to THE KING, and as he turned back, the cloaked person was gone.

The Queen quickly approached the King, reaching out to see what the King was given. As the Queen pulled back the cloth in the basket, she and the King heard a whimper…and then a coo. A child appeared, a baby! Both the King and the Queen gasped and continued to look around, expecting to see the cloaked person, but he was nowhere to be found.

The Queen looked at the King and said, "This child has eyes that are not like ours, his hands seem different, and his face is different as well" The King paused…

"We will take in this child and raise him until the cloaked person returns." And so the Queen bent down to their Princess and introduced her to the new Prince.

Days, months, and even years had gone by, and the King and Queen raised the small child as their own. Proudly accepting the prince's differences, as he was slow to learn, slow to take part in activities, and even slow to speak. The Kingdom also accepted the Prince as one of their own, and he eventually grew to shine a brilliant light of kindness, caring, and a smile that provided unmatched love to anyone who witnessed it. The Prince was a gift not only to the King and Queen but to the entire Kingdom.

Many, many years later, as the King, Queen, Princess, and Prince were outside the Kingdom's great walls enjoying time together, playing in the afternoon sunset, an image appeared to be walking towards them…it caught the King's attention. The King turned toward the approaching person, blinded somewhat by the brilliance of the setting sun, directly behind the person. As the shadow got closer, the King began to recognize…it was the cloaked person who many years ago brought the Prince to the King.

"Good day," said the mysterious person as he kept his head down, so to not let the King see who he was. The King, in turn, wished the traveler welcome.

The King asked, "What can I do for you today, my friend?" as the Prince began to walk just beside the King, attaching himself to the King's hip.

"Do you not remember me… I once told you I would return and so I am here." The King stood stoic, recalling what the cloaked person said those many years ago. "I must ask you again," said the cloaked man, "are you a good person?" The King paused…this time recalling the man's suggestion that he would lose everything had he not changed his ways.

The King continued to ponder his response and then said to the man in a soulful manner, "Please come meet my family, the Queen, the Princess, and my son the Prince…they can answer your question." With that the cloaked man raised up his head to show his brilliant smile as though he was satisfied, happy with the King's introduction of the Prince.

With that slight gesture, the visitor faded away with the remaining bit sunlight, exclaiming, "You truly are a good person and a good family…there is nothing you will ever lose as long as you have each other."

The moral to this story…accept gifts, no matter the package it comes in, no matter the challenges you might experience, and share it with the world, and it can never be taken from you and will only make you better through the love you share and the work you do to build your happiness.

About This Book

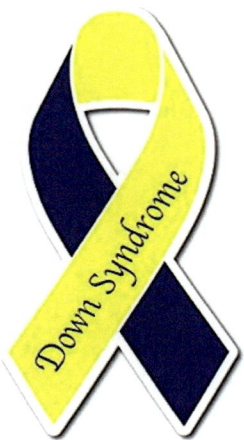

We didn't know…what we didn't know…

We'd like to introduce you to our handsome son Logan. As you get to know Logan and our family through reading about our "normal life," we want you to know our hearts were once shocked with a completely unexpected diagnosis, which eventually became the foundation of our lives.

As you read further, know, as overwhelming as it may seem, you have now taken your first step through a door to an unbiased life and unexpected happiness, not of panic or fear as most tend to think.

There is help and support out there; you just need to know where to look for it. The doubt and fear of the unknown you feel right now is something we can assure you subsides the moment you hold your swaddled, new baby, look into their bright eyes, and say hello for the first time. We can only hope our story can help provide you comfort, knowing your journey begins with the love you share with your new baby and how it is, in-turn, shared, making the world a better place.

On day one…our hearts jump into our throats, our minds began to scramble uncontrollably, the news absolutely took our breath away, and we couldn't begin to know what to do or feel. The emotional distress, which was never expected, very quickly launched us both into another layer of reality, where it felt like there is no one to help and not one book to guide you through this new and unexpected journey. Remember, Google and YouTube weren't even in their infancy, and we were desperate to know if our love was strong enough to support one another during this truly shocking time. "What do we do?" runs through our whole family's mindset for years to come. The answer most times is simple, BREATHE..."You will love EACH OTHER." There's a new normal ahead, you will get there.

Looking back, the day Logan was born, his birth was absolutely "normal."

Other than a thirty-five-week premature labor, we expected nothing to be concerned with until the nurses, while bathing him, picked up some genetic markers and our doctor told us they needed to run some tests on our son. Albeit nearly twenty years ago, the moment, a frozen memory in time, "seems like it was just yesterday." Processing this information can only be compared to the shock of losing your dreams, your "ideal," your "normal," the dream you built as a child of finding your Prince, building your very own family and living your perfect "happily ever after."

As a parent, you immediately grieve for the "ideal baby" you lost and don't know how to process the void of your dream and the new and unexpected diagnosis. The amount of time the grieving process takes is different with each individual, each family, and you will go through all five steps, ending with acceptance.

STOP! Take a BREATH and tell yourself, "YOU GOT THIS"...because YOU DO...it may not seem like it right away, but we're writing this FOR YOU, to assure you YOU DO! You have just received a WONDERFUL GIFT, just like any other child. BREATHE and just wait...be patient, you will see!

Through these years of raising a baby, then a child, then young adult with special needs (for us Down syndrome), the experiences you have and the people you meet and befriend, may not be what you expected as a young couple, but it's up to you to redefine your expectations and JUST BE A PARENT and enjoy the unconditional love your family has just received. This may not be the road you planned, but you will certainly enjoy this journey.

We can only hope this book provides you what we did not have; experience, knowledge, and even hope, knowing a child with special needs, although exhausting at times, is really not much different than any other son or daughter, just a different pace of life.

The ignorance of the past, the stereotypes, and the cultural misgivings seem to never go away. It's up to all of us to educate the world of the unique and very special life we have experienced, as you will soon see.

You will read not only our own personal experience but the clinical and educational benefits and struggles we have worked through with Logan, his teachers, schools, and the community as a whole.

Welcome to the SPECIAL FAMILIES CLUB; embark on this journey knowing we are all here to help! Friends don't let friends count chromosomes. We are all Down Right Normal.

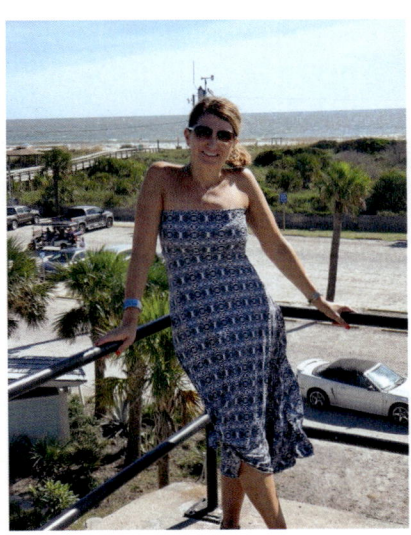 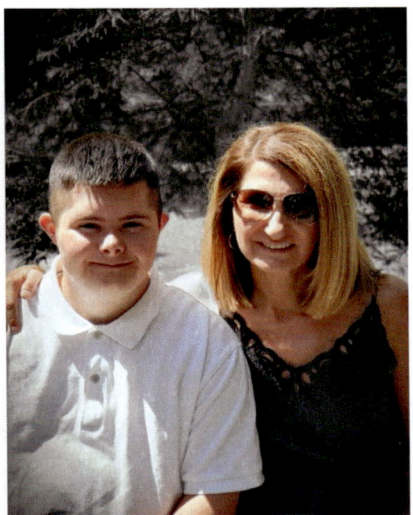

Foreword

by Dr. Monica LaPore,

Professor West Chester University, Kinesiology Department

My first awareness of Down syndrome came in an awkward moment in my neighborhood in New York City when I was a teenager. As my mom and I walked toward church, I glanced down a side block where I saw our family friend helping a young man, about my age, out of a car in front of their apartment building. When I inquired to my mom who the young man was, she glanced down the block, quickly turned her head to look straight ahead, and kept walking briskly toward our destination. I was shocked that not only did she not answer me, but she did not shout out a greeting and a wave to her friend.

It was a quiet Sunday morning in fall 1974, and I was a college student studying to be a teacher. I was at a curious and introspective stage of my life at which I was discovering a whole other world existed outside my neighborhood, outside of my small circle of tight-knit family and friends. I was excited to be learning about educational concepts and theories in college classes so that I could one day become a teacher. I was interested in mysteries of the world, notions that were far-off from my over-protected life, and people and places that would give me pause.

It was more than curious that my mom did not answer my question regarding the young man, so I asked again. Her answer was the beginning of my deep reflections on what it means for others to view someone as "different" and what it might mean to care about someone with a visible difference. My mom finally told me that the young man had Down syndrome, was the son of her friend, and lived in an "institution." I was shocked! I had been at the home of this family many times, and no one mentioned a son who lived somewhere else. *What does that mean?* I thought. *Why did he not live with his family?* Thus began a true longing to understand the lives of people with Down syndrome, their families, and their friends.

Fast forward forty years and I have the privilege to meet Logan Patterson and his family. Logan lives with Down syndrome and became a member of my Special Olympics soccer, basketball, and swim teams as a teenager. Logan is a wonderful young man who loves basketball, dancing, friends, and is rocking his transition program. He and his family joined our "Rammie's family," a group of over forty families who put their heart and soul into supporting three sports teams of individuals with intellectual disabilities who love and care for each other. Shortly after meeting Logan, I discovered that his mom, Cheryl, was writing daily Facebook posts throughout the month of October (Down syndrome awareness month) to debunk myths, provide facts, and provide hope and education to individuals with Down syndrome, their families and friends, support personnel, potential employers, and policymakers. Cheryl's daily Down syndrome posts encouraged me to look beyond medical diagnosis, stereotypes, and labels and to view the underlying aspects of Down syndrome as only part of the big picture of life with Logan and his friends.

After more than forty years of advocating, supporting, and befriending many individuals with Down syndrome, I am excited to introduce this book to you, from the eyes of a loving, caring, always-advocating mom who wants the world to give her son— and all individuals with Down syndrome— an equitable opportunity of living, loving, working, recreating, and learning in the same places as we all live, love, work, and learn.

Monica Lepore

Day 1

The Best Life, Promise!

Often when a child is born with Down syndrome, doctors accompany the news with an "I'm sorry…" They may throw out a bunch of facts, figures, and medical jargon, creating one, overwhelming experience for a new parent. It's certainly not the way to welcome a new life into the world, especially one that is your child.

So what's the right thing to tell a new parent of a child with Down syndrome? How about **"Congratulations?"** (Themighty.com) After all they are still your child.

Logan attended Camp Pals (a sleep away camp) since the age of sixteen, and one of the activities during the week long sleep away camp is The **Congratulations** Project.

This project enables the CAMPERS to work with their Camp Buddies (Counselors) to write letters to new parents who have given birth to a baby with Down syndrome. Here are some samples from the Congratulation letters….AMAZING

My name is (John, Jane, Lizzy or even Logan)…and I was born with Down syndrome…

"P.S. This baby is going to be the best thing that ever happens to you."

"Good luck with your baby. Don't be scared. Be happy because they are going to be great and successful."

"Your baby will have a wonderful life like mine. Please don't be scared. Down syndrome is amazing."

Friends don't let friend's count chromosomes ♥

#friendsdon'tletfriendscountchromosomes #specialneedsmom #downsyndrome #downsyndromeawareness #proudmom #selfadvocate #personfirstlanguage #therock #dwaynjohnson #markwahlberg #normalisboring #diversity #siblings #target

Day 2

How to Say Things When You Don't Know What to Say

Eloquence does not come to everyone naturally, no matter their status, their level of education, or their social standing; some say the gifts of eloquence and empathy are shaped through living the experience and placing yourself in the shoes of others.

As a new special family, you will hear various different ways of phrasing things; be patient, take a step back and realize others have not lived your experience and the grace you provide, more times than not, will help fill your soul with pride, pride you never experienced before, the pride of knowing you have helped another improve their lack of understanding in the world today, you, my friend, become the teacher.

We have found having a child with special needs opens you up to a number of opportunities you would never thought you had experienced, like being an interpreter.

For instance most moms and dads understand the early stages of babble and have to interpret what their child is saying, sometimes for other family members. In the case of our doctor, interpretation should have never been something we needed and yet his explanation and "guidance" took on a whole other meaning. In the haze of confusion, we didn't know how to interpret what he was attempting to explain to us, and as a result, frustration grew exponentially.

Over time you begin to understand words not only have definition but to some degree hidden meaning behind them. Feelings of uncertainty, confusion, or sadness come to you, not because what just happened but through the friends and family who don't know what to say. You are quickly launched into the realm of sympathy, empathy, and to some degree sadness but need to understand words become difficult for you and your loved ones to express.

As you begin to develop a sensitive ear, you'll need to absorb the words, understand them in a different way, and always look at things from ALL SIDES.

Ying has Yang, Good has Bad, and you now have the gift of balance, but only if you see, or in this case hear, things from both sides.

Friends don't let friend's count chromosomes ♥

#friendsdon'tletfriendscountchromosomes #specialneedsmom #downsyndrome #downsyndromeawareness #proudmom #selfadvocate #personfirstlanguage

Day 3

Why "Down" Syndrome

Down syndrome, believe it or not, is not a negative connotation passed from one generation to another. Prior to what we know today as Down syndrome, a Psychologist coined a clinical definition in 1910 as "Moron," which today takes on a whole different meaning. "Moron" was simply a way to describe someone as having a mental perspective of between seven and ten years of age.

Down syndrome is actually named after the English doctor, John Langdon Down, who in 1866 was the first to categorize the common features of people with what came to be later understood as a genetic variation.

What if a child is born with Down syndrome instead of the doctor saying, "Your child has a chromosome abnormality," the doctor used different adjectives, maybe "Your child was born with Down syndrome, which is a genetic variation or an alternative genetic arrangement." This sounds less "moronic" (in today's terms) and certainly better than abnormality. In our eyes, there is nothing abnormal here.

Friends don't let friend's count chromosomes ♥

#friendsdon'tletfriendscountchromosomes #specialneedsmom #downsyndrome #downsyndromeawareness #proudmom #selfadvocate #personfirstlanguage

Day 4

No Judgment

I always tell friends and family my house is a "judgment free zone."

No one knows what goes on behind closed doors. No one truly knows their journey, and while they may share it with a select few, sharing a story and living it are two different realities.

You can empathize, support, and even lend an ear...honestly be prepared...you'll need it often. My journey is different, as is everyone else's, it's unique to each of us, but it's no less beautiful, stressful, love-filled crazy! Remember, everyone has something, and I love all of my something's.

Friends don't let friend's count chromosomes ❤

#friendsdon'tletfriendscountchromosomes #specialneedsmom #downsyndrome #downsyndromeawareness #proudmom #selfadvocate

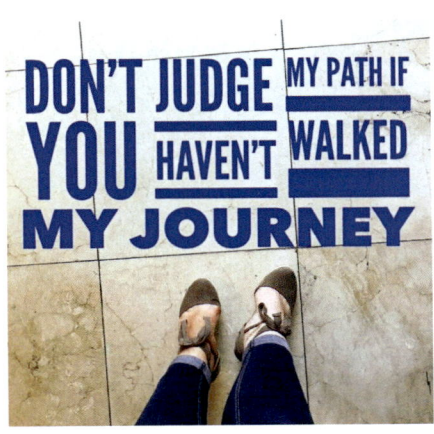

Confronting Ignorance

Expect to be confronted with the "R word" (retarded) at some point. We look at it this way, each generation, every race, almost every belief has come under the guise of judgment, judgment based in ignorance more times than not. So we had a choice, become angry and hateful, like those who chose the path of ignorance, or rise above and use what you now know as the better path and educate those who do not know and make them sensitive to others.

Approach it like this, "…let me ask you a question…you are probably more familiar with the N-word, right? Would you loosely use the N-word in a public setting where others within ears' reach could hear you? How do you think you come across to those around you when you use a word like that? … I just heard you mention a word that is more commonly used in the wrong way and is just as offensive as the N-word, it's known as the R-word. Is there a better word you can use, or maybe think about how you would feel if someone used a personally demeaning word to describe you?"

Expect a very uncomfortable, chattering response of, "Oh…I'm sorry, I wasn't talking about you or your son/daughter," where you cordially respond, "I understand…just know there are folks who are very hurt by what you just said and there are better ways to describe someone you feel may not be as smart, understanding, and warm hearted as you."

Day 5

It's About the Journey

Progress - forward or onward movement toward a destination.

Logan's development, although slow, has definitely progressed over the years. I sometimes feel like we are stagnant but then I find some little treasure that shows me otherwise.

Today cleaning out bins in the basement, I found Logan's weekend book from the 2011/2012 school year. As I sat there and paged through his book, I am reminded of how far we have come and at what rate doesn't really matter.

Celebrate EVERY little accomplishment, no matter how small. I'm not sure of the destination, but I'm enjoying our journey. I stated previously that Logan and other children with delays hit their milestones at different rates.

Friends don't let friend's count chromosomes ♥

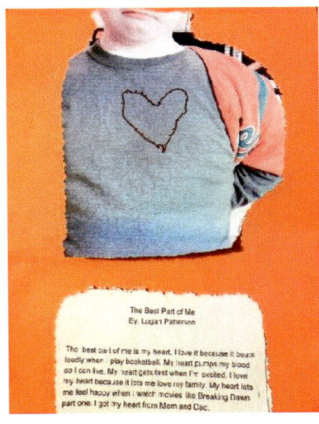

Day 6

Setting Expectations

Parents of children with Down syndrome are given limitations, expectation "norms" from the day their children are born, and in some cases prior. We are told there is a Down syndrome growth chart, most children have long-term (chronic) constipation problems. Sleep apnea (because the mouth, throat, and airway are narrowed in children with Down syndrome), teeth that appear later than normal and in a location that may cause problems with chewing or not appear at all (maybe missing adult teeth).

Underactive thyroid (hypothyroidism), low muscle tone, poor judgment, low attention span, slow learning, eye problems, hip problems (medlineplus.gov) among others. They will need long-term care, never live on their own, hold a job, have a meaningful life.

While some of these are true of Logan, the realization of these expectations you are given at birth is overwhelming to say the least

IF YOU CANNOT PREDICT HER FUTURE, PLEASE STOP TRYING TO PREDICT HIS.

Friends don't let friend's count chromosomes ♥

What to Expect

Go ahead…jump from website to website…asking the question, what should I expect? Expect NOTHING and make your child's future the best it can be. Each child is unique with or without needs. Let each child "be" whoever they want.

Remember earlier when I said BREATHE… You can drive yourself crazy looking for the ever-elusive crystal ball. If it existed, we would all have it. So let's walk through some of what you will find and will unnecessarily worry about and we are going to tell you to STOP, just STOP!

Below are some of the common things you can expect to hear, but we can assure you it is not one size fits all. There is balance throughout life and the captions you see throughout the internet are nothing more than panic mongering because it's easier to fall into the negative of ANY situation, so we thought we would balance it out the negative with what we have witnessed firsthand:

WHAT YOU WILL FIND	WHAT ACTUALLY HAPPENS
Your baby will have heart problems	The reported incidence of Congenital Heart Disease is between 40-60%. Commonly described as a defect; the most common being an AVSD (www.ncbi.nlm.nih.gov). Logan had a VSD at birth that spontaneously closed by age two, and he was discharged from cardiology.
Your baby likely won't walk until 3yrs	SO WHAT...patience is a virtue, walking will come when the time is right...worry more about toilet training ;-) Our experience with Logan you ask? He never crawled, he went from scooting to walking.
Your baby is likely to have cancer	Children with DS have an increased risk for acute lymphoblastic leukemia than children born without DS. Any child can be diagnosed with cancer just like any adult; don't stress over things we cannot control. Watch for signs, like petechiae, Logan used to get this rash when he had a virus. At first I thought he had leukemia the moment I saw it, but it was just how his body reacts to being sick with a virus. You will know when something is off, trust your instinct.
Your child won't make friends	Again this can be true DS or not. It will be up to you to sign your child up for typical and special Olympic/Challenger league activities. A combination of these activities will make your child feel accepted. You will know what is best, follow your intuition on what your child needs and likes. I never liked basketball, but due to a bond between Logan and an elementary school friend, Logan excelled in basketball as a high school team manager and in Special Olympics.
Send your child away to a home	This is mostly an "old school" thought, and thank goodness, is not thought of much today. Most children flourish in their home environment, and because of this change in mind set, the life expectancy of individuals with Down syndrome has dramatically increased.

Day 7

Advocating from the Heart

I often ask myself why I advocate. It's not my personality; I would be content flying under the radar. This has been my personality FOREVER and still is on most topics. For almost twenty-one years, when I entered into motherhood, almost nineteen years ago when I entered into the special needs community, I found my voice for many reasons. I advocate for:

Education - Most people, I believe, just need education to have some understanding in order to make good decisions. Most people are scared of the unknown.

Strive, Beyond Your Comfort Zone – Logan, who has the same rights as his typical peers, with things as simple as attending a dance or as complicated as education and employment.

Understanding – Helping people to be aware there is a significant connotation of the "R-word" or any demeaning language that society has grown numb to over the last several decades

Role models - Speak up, stand up for people who cannot, if not me, who would? Be the good.

Advocate Love

Advocate is defined as a person who publicly supports or recommends a particular cause or policy (Oxford Dictionary).

We are all advocates in one way or another. Advocating is the parental instinct of knowing what is right for your child with or without needs and telling someone about it.

When any child is born, they NEED us to advocate for them, to speak up on their behalf and tell friends, therapists, doctors, anyone who will listen what they need. We as parents know what is best for our children and know them best. Now add in your child has special needs, and you need to advocate that much louder.

As your child ages, just like any other child, we want them to learn to express their needs and wants and advocate for themselves. It could be something as simple as what they want to eat, or to expressing their feelings about a situation. This is a learned and mimicked trait we need to instill in all our children.

Friends don't let friend's count chromosomes ❤

#friendsdontletfriendscountchromosomes #target #specialneedsmom #advocate #downsyndromeawareness #proudmom #selfadvocate #personfirstlanguage #therock #dwaynjohnson #markwahlberg #normalisboring #diversity #siblings #theluckyfew #downsyndrome

Day 8

Finding Your Tribe

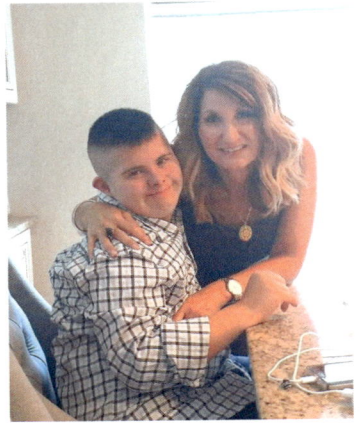

Making friends after forty feels almost impossible, then add in a child with special needs and it feels even more unimaginable. You are understandably exhausted. It feels like you can't relate to anyone anymore and no one can relate to you.

I can't even tell you how wonderful it is when you find people that understand and take the time to truly listen. I am beyond lucky that I have a supportive "tribe" of friends and family that not only listen to me but spend time with Logan as well.

Start your own "Especially Hot Momma's Club" or "Dads' Down Pack."

It's amazing when it happens, but getting there is hard. I am one blessed, lucky women.

To my tribe, you know who you are, I couldn't take this journey without you.

Friends don't let friend's count chromosomes ♥

#friendsdon'tletfriendscountchromosomes #specialneedsmom #downsyndrome #downsyndromeawareness #proudmom #mytribe

Day 9

Best Friends Forever

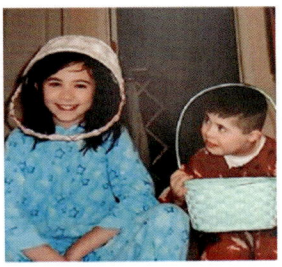

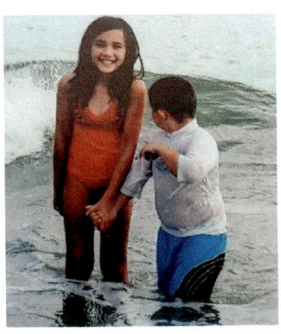

While having a sibling with Down syndrome may present unique challenges (https://www.ndss.org), it also provides many opportunities for children's positive growth and character development on both sides of the fence. I was initially anxious for Kayla, our daughter, Logan's big sister, regarding the effect of having a brother with Down syndrome.

Contrary to my anxieties, I believe it has had positive impacts on their relationship. Kayla tends to be more aware of the difficulties, others might be going through. Having Logan as a sibling has shaped not only her personality but her decisions in life.

She has routinely volunteered for Special Olympics, joined Alpha Sigma Alpha sorority because they raise money and support Special Olympics, as well as just being an all around great, loving sister.

Love these pictures and the way Logan looks up to Kayla, especially when he was little. She will be most likely be his longest relationship in life. I am so happy they have each other.

Day 10

Don't Change a Thing

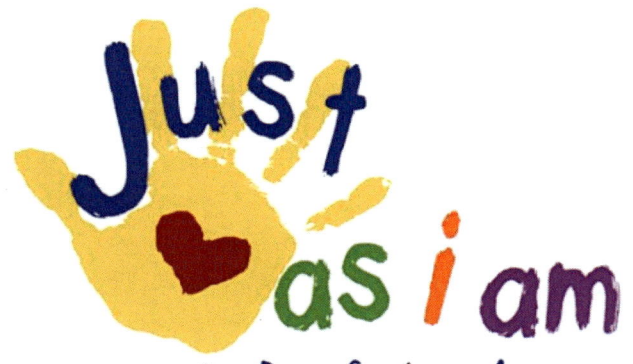

supporting Down Syndrome Awareness

I have been asked, "What if Logan didn't have Down syndrome, or what if they could cure it?"

Here's what we would've missed out on over the last nineteen years if Logan didn't have Down syndrome.:

- Logan's sensitivity to others emotions, his true sensitivity to show empathy toward others.
- Knowing true success is not measured by your income level or education, it is measured by how you treat others in this life. Choose kind!
- Learning more life lessons from him than I have taught him in more than nineteen years of life, which in turn has truly made me a better person.
- The beauty in differences in ALL people.

- Appreciate everything, no matter how small. Every accomplishment, every joyful moment, every minute of every day.
- Celebrate diversity, there is no "normal."

Just a few things I would have truly missed, there are many more I could list. Logan is our true teacher in life and I am a better person for it. Don't live in the world of...IF!

Get Out of Your Own Head

Being where you are now, we can assure you "you don't know what you don't know"...so our advice is NOT to over think things, get out of your own head, and enjoy the life experience you are living.

Over these nineteen years of being a special family, we have used what we learned being a parent of our beautiful daughter to be better parents for both her and Logan. Life is the ultimate learning experience.

This is all new for you as much as it was for us, as it is for all families typical or not. After some time, if you decide to use this book as a learning experience, you begin to see things differently from a completely different perspective... and before you know it, you see the goodness in all things. It's up to you to apply it to the relationships you have with your friends, family, colleagues, and acquaintances.

As you go out, providing your son/daughter with life's experiences, you will begin to bond with other special families. Some of your child's best friends might have Down syndrome, Autism, Cerebral Palsy, or other various physical, mental, emotional challenges, or no challenges at all. Either one and all are OK. You will see, learn, and lean on them more than you ever thought was capable.

At first these challenges may seem somewhat overwhelming. Look at it this way; go back to when you were a small child during your shy time, when your parents introduced you to a stranger for the first time, you clung to your mother's leg, turning your head away from this extraordinarily large person, who at first was intimidating. As the days, months, and even years went by, you eventually came to call this person Uncle or Aunt or a close friend of your parents.

Just like you are getting used to your favorite aunt, working with children with various challenges may feel unsettled at first. Watching a child with Down syndrome "shut down" and refuse to move from the ground they are sitting on or witnessing a child with Autism become physical with themselves as a result of frustration or over stimulation from the sounds you don't even notice, eventually the shock factor subsides, just like it did when you got to know your aunt. This will be your new "normal."

Just know...don't over think the situation or reaction, it is your child trying to communicate, and they may be frustrated since they are unable to tell you in the same way you understand.. YOU have done nothing wrong, they have done nothing wrong, PATIENCE with one another and knowing this moment is temporary and greater understanding is yet to come.

Day 11

Bonding Family, Bonding Community

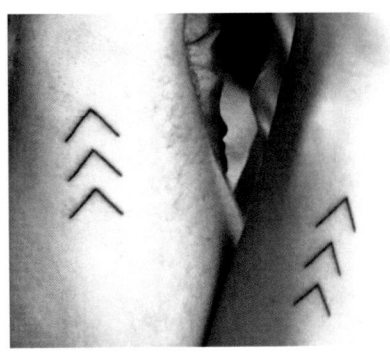

Logan has ALWAYS wanted a tattoo. He loves Dwayne Johnson, Mark Wahlberg, and his Pee-Pop's tattoos. A few years ago, Kayla wanted a tattoo and I decided I would go with her and get a Down syndrome tattoo for Logan.

There is a tattoo called the lucky few. A group of mothers who had children with Down syndrome were at a retreat and decided they wanted a tattoo to bond them together that was full of meaning. They settled on a design of three simple arrows in a row. "The three arrows symbolize the three twenty-first chromosomes and how we rise up and move forward. We fly the highest after we have been pulled back and stretched, sometimes even more than we think we can bear" (https://themighty.com/.../.../parents-kids-down-syndrome-tattoo/).

I decided this was perfect for my first and only tattoo. Many parents have followed since then, including siblings, grandparents, extended family, and close friends. All united by loving someone with Down syndrome.

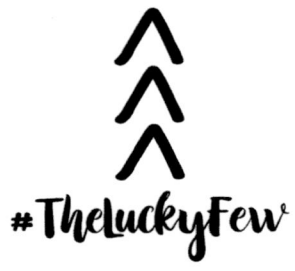

The Inseparable Bond
Siblings

There was life before Logan. Kayla, was born January 1st, 1999. Kayla was our first born; she was perfect, all six pounds, four ounces, twenty-one inches long and at thirty-five weeks! Like any other typical child, she met her milestones, and we celebrated each and every one.

Kayla was an only child for 717 days until December 18th, 2000 at thirty-five weeks, just like his sister, Logan Patrick entered the world. He was only slightly smaller than Kayla, five pounds, fifteen ounces, and nineteen inches long but no less mighty.

The moment Kayla met her brother, she was in love. She mothered him from day one. When Logan was home and getting his therapies, Kayla helped. She watched over him fiercely. Kayla is now twenty-one and Logan nineteen, and at times there has definitely been a role reversal of sorts.

Logan likes to watch over his sister, worries about her, and misses her, even when she is gone as little as an hour. Logan has, as long as I can remember and still does, look up to his sister as his protector, for advice, for fun, and hugs. I love their bond and everything about it.

Logan's natural ability to form attachments is unique. There has been no pattern to who he attaches to, but once he forms his bond, it is unbreakable. There are some family members, teachers, family friends, and our church Deacon to name a few.

Teachers

Let's be honest, teachers, of all studies, are overwhelmingly underpaid and underappreciated for the work they do. Teachers guide the next stages of their students' lives; some special needs teachers themselves rise above an already exceptional group of humans.

The patience and parent-like protective bond some of these worldly angels wrap around our children is a grace unmatched. Our fellow special parents whose hearts swell knowing there are others who understand and not only guide our children but guide us as well. The teachers you will encounter, some better than others, some will be exceptional, provide the light of hope, shining a light on your truly unique child, unique in ways you never expected.

Since we are speaking of bonds, know this, the bond between your child and some of their teachers can only be matched by the bond of teacher and parent, and it is up to you to fortify that bond, if not for your child, for you and your spouse. This teacher/parent bond can be limitless, priceless resource that follows your son or daughter throughout their lives.

If we talk about the bond of teachers, we can't get away without mentioning fellow students. We think of Logan's fellow elementary students as siblings from another house. Funny, I know, but you'll see throughout this book while also learning from many other families, the bond between children will impact our childrens' lives, from the food they eat, to the sports they play, to most of their social behaviors.

Friends

No matter where we go, within three miles or 500 miles, we inevitably always run into someone who says, "…is that Logan?" In King's Dominion (in Virginia) or Disney World (Florida), in a local café or on the beach, Logan is the very famous (some might say infamous), unofficial mayor of our little sleepy 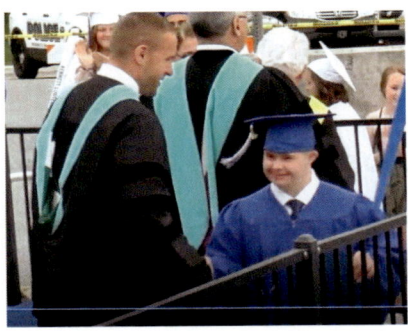 town. The level of excitement people approach us with when they see Logan outside the environment they share with him shows us the level to which Logan can make an impact on a life.

Heartwarming does not begin to measure this insatiable feeling, one I wish I could say I experienced as a child. This bond Logan creates, as I am sure your special child will also create, found its crescendo during his high school graduation.

Just imagine more than 400 students waiting to hear their names being read by their principal to rush the stage, to receive their diploma they fought so hard for eighteen years to receive and the cheers they received from their four to five family members who were able to attend, since there were limited tickets for each student to keep the crowds under control during this event, also applause was to be kept to the end of the presentation for time purposes. You hear Michael Shaw, Betty Jane Masterson, Juan Alverez...LOGAN PATTERSON (the ONLY loudly exaggerated name read by the Vice Principal) and the AUDIENCE, students, and families alike ARUPT in applause, as though you were at the final fourth and two play of the Super Bowl. Totally unexpected! But this is what you build within your child through yourself, the parents you meet, the teachers you work with, and the students who grow to love your child as a fellow classmate/friend.

#friendsdon'tletfriendscountchromosomes #specialneedsmom #downsyndrome #downsyndromeawareness #proudmom #selfadvocate #personfirstlanguage #therock #dwaynjohnson #markwahlberg #normalisboring #diversity #siblings #theluckyfew

Day 12

Their Favorites

Logan, like other kids, LOVES his grand-parents fiercely and unconditionally.

Logan has a special bond with each one, from having coffee with Grammie (when he should have been drinking milk), having spam with Pop-Pop for breakfast (because he never had it at home), to making up songs about Disney and getting pet names from Mee-Mom and Pee-Pop like "Grasshopper" and "Log-on."

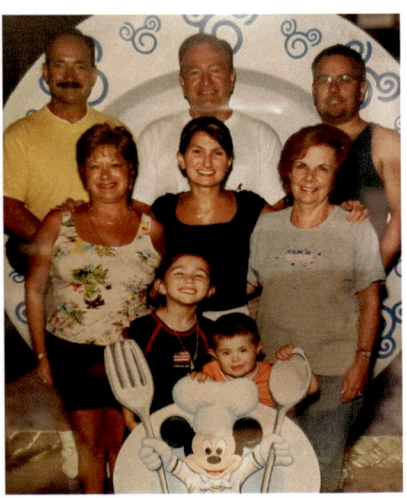

When his Mee-Mom and Pop-Pop were sick and eventually passed, it was and is such a hard concept for him to grasp. His empathy for our parents while they were sick was heartwarming and heartbreaking all at the same time to say the least.

Logan had problems relaying his feelings as a pre-teen and teen. He never cried out of sadness or pain or verbally expressed distress until his two grand-parents passed. He cried and still does on occasion, and that's OK.

Friends don't let friend's count chromosomes ♥

#therock #dwaynjohnson #markwahlberg #normalisboring #diversity #siblings #grandparents

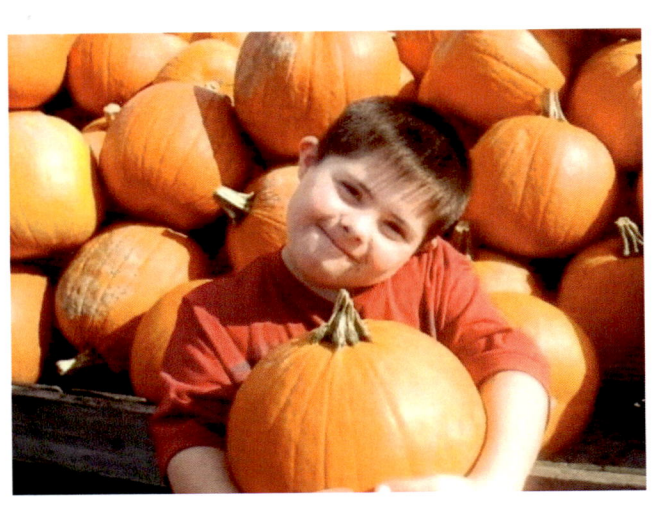

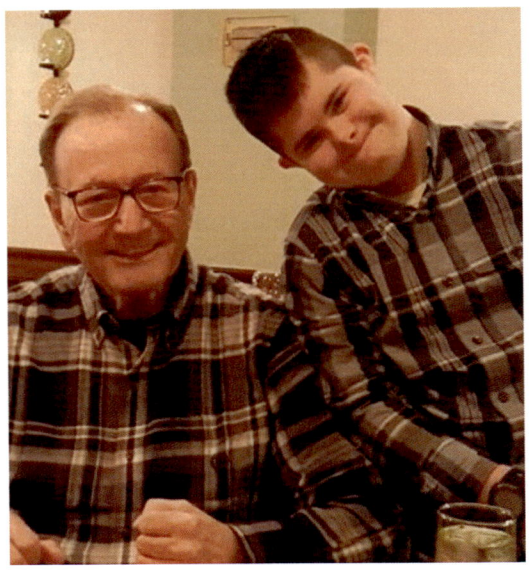

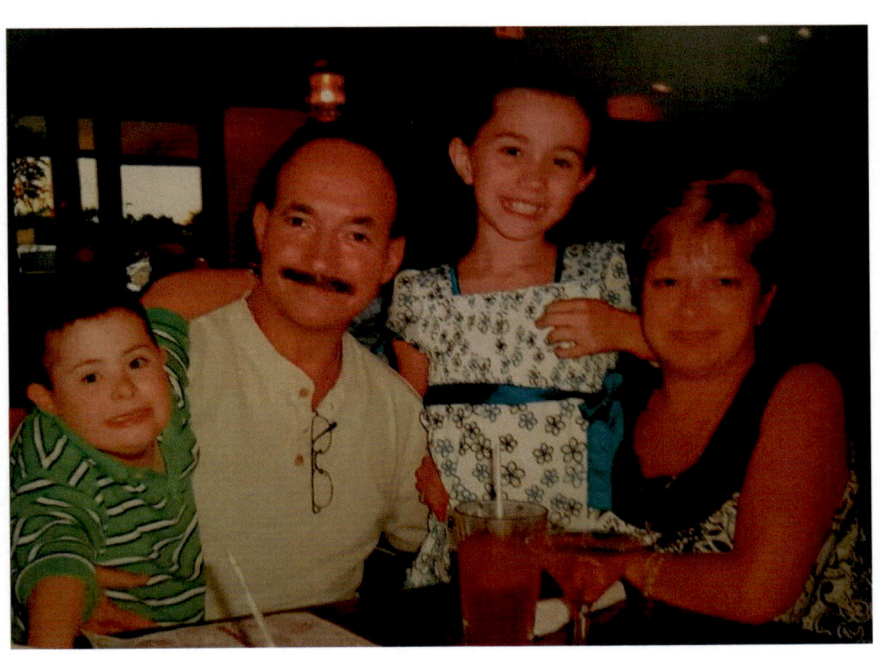

Sensitive Subjects

Now the tough conversations; yes, your special child or young adult will have emotional connections throughout their lives and the loss of a connection, like any of us, is devastating.

We dare not suggest what you should or should not do in times of family illness or death. Living through two extreme diagnosis of cancer with two teenagers, Kayla and Logan, it is hard for both to grasp why their grandparent can't walk outside with them, can't make them breakfast anymore, and eventually can't tell them they love them because they lost their ability to speak; it is an experience we so desperately wish we could take away, but it is a factor of life.

From the time Logan was a toddler, we would hear him talking in his room to himself, or so we thought. Into adolescence and pre-teen years, it continued. Write it off as creative imagination, but we began to have other considerations.

The amount of unconditional love Logan brings into this world is truly unique; your child may be no different. The change that naturally happens as their lives touch your family, your friends, and well beyond throughout their entire lives, and what seems to be the ability to see only good is BEYOND SPECIAL, almost how life was meant to be.

We could not help but feel Logan brings the gift of himself into this world and maintains a connection, as a gift to them, to guardians he only sees and hears.

You may witness this overwhelming experience in some way. It's as hard to explain as it is to believe, but even now at the age of nineteen years, Logan comes to me out of the blue and says, "Pop-Pop said to say hi," and even without asking, Logan took his Mee-Mom's urn to his room and said she wanted to stay with him in his room. A chill runs down your spine as you realize there is truly a connection of some kind and their ability or inability grasp the concept of death IS NOT because they don't understand it, it's just the opposite, they clearly understand the connection more than most of us because it is and always will be part of who they are.

Mee-Mom and Pop-Pop are always there for Logan, and he can't see it any other way. We believe the extra chromosome is a bridge beyond what we as parents or typical kids may experience during our lives. That bridge allows Logan's guardian to remain in touch with him, guide him, and show us how to be better people.

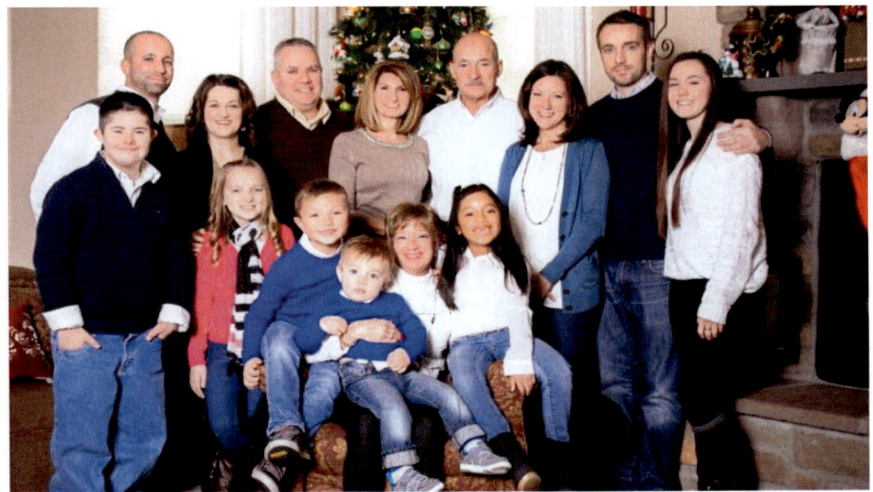

Day 13

Medical Considerations

Many children born with Down syndrome have no serious medical complications but some will. The most common is hearing loss. Three-quarters of people with Down syndrome have hearing difficulties (Healthline.com).

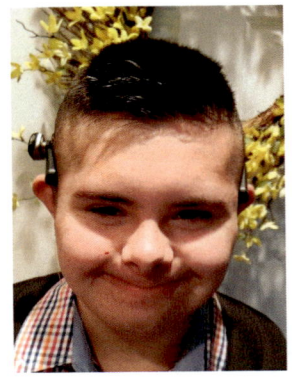

When Logan was born, we didn't know of his Down syndrome diagnosis. Logan does have hearing loss. Logan has had twelve ear surgeries from the age of two to sixteen years, and chances are we are not done yet. Ten of the ear surgeries were for drainage tubes, but during the last surgery while they were placing tubes, they found a tumor behind his right ear drum called a cholesteotoma (which is benign). They went back in two months later, and after a four hour surgery, it was removed.

Logan's hearing loss did not improve post surgery as we had hoped, so a year ago, May 2018, he received a BAHA bone vibrating hearing aide. He sees an audiologist on a routine basis to test his hearing and still see ENT every two months to have them remove debris from his ears. If you ask him about surgery, he will tell you he LOVES the sleep part, with a smile of course. Logan is still rocking that hearing aide look.

Friends don't let friend's count chromosomes ♥

Consider this

It's important for parents not be afraid to ask questions to other adults and kids alike when you see something you don't understand; ask about it respectfully.

All our children are little sponges, and when they see something that is different, it's appropriate to start a conversation; don't be afraid to instill the interest of educating for one's self instead of avoiding differences.

Logan wears his hearing aide everyday to school and certain functions outside of school. Yes, it makes him stand out amongst the majority who don't wear devices. If you were to introduce yourself, Logan would gladly tell you what it is, and before you know it, Logan is your best new friend.

Logan's a trooper, and it really doesn't seem to bother him in the least, as with most of life, he lets it roll off his back. An example most of us can learn as adults.

Day 14

Signs

A single transverse palmar crease (also known as Simian crease) is a single crease that extends across the palm of the hand, formed by the fusion of the two palmar creases and is found in people with Trisomy 18 and Trisomy 21 (Down syndrome)

Approximately 45% of people with Down syndrome have a single palmer crease. This is the result of hypotonia, as the hand was not held in a tight fist as they were growing in utero (this was a new fact for me).

Logan has one hand with a Simian crease and one without, as did his grandfather. A family genetic trait or Trisomy 21 trait, to this day, we don't exactly know.

Logan's decreased tone (hypotonia) is challenging for him to perform fine motor skills, like writing, tying his shoe, buttons, and performing some self care. His determination more than makes up for his low tone.

Friends don't let friend's count chromosomes ♥

#friendsdon'tletfriendscountchromosomes #specialneedsmom #downsyndrome #downsyndromeawareness #proudmom #selfadvocate #personfirstlanguage

Consider This – Apgar, Signs they look for

A large number of people with and without Down syndrome have a Simian crease. There are certain characteristics/traits of Down syndrome they look for after birth. Simian crease is only one of them. Individuals with Down syndrome have an array of traits that is unique to them.

The Apgar test, the medical test nurses administer minutes after every birth, takes into consideration physical attributes including lower set ears, extra skin on the back of the neck, first and second toe separation, and almond shaped eyes to name some.

Let's remember these are traits of Down syndrome, your child will still have Grandpa's eye color, Auntie's hair color and curls, Mom's nose, along with a million other little idiosyncrasies and traits that are unique to you and your family. After a while, you will not "see" the Down syndrome traits. I know I don't with Logan. I see Logan.

Day 15

Finding the Right Fit

Children and adults with Down syndrome have a unique body habitus. They start with lower birth rates, and some struggle with significant medical problems in their first days of life, therefore delaying their growth.

Logan's body habitus is different from other young adults his age, which has made it incredibly difficult over the years to find clothing to fit him properly and still be in "style." Logan's short stature, increased waist circumference, and low tone are a challenge with pants and other clothing with different fasteners. Shoes are also a challenge when shopping due to Logan's, wide toe box, flat arch, and small feet.

Kudos to Target, Tommy Hilfiger, and Nike, to mention a few, for supplying clothing and shoes that are age appropriate and stylish for our children. Hopefully other retailers will follow suit, as this line makes it less stressful for parents to find proper fitting clothes that our young adults feel comfortable and stylish in.

Friends don't let friend's count chromosomes ♥

#friendsdon'tletfriendscountchromosomes #specialneedsmom #downsyndrome #downsyndromeawareness #proudmom #selfadvocate #personfirstlanguage #therock #dwaynjohnson #markwahlberg

You got a friend in me
The aforementioned therapies and their importance carry us through all aspects and ages of growth for our children.

Let's talk about getting dressed; from pulling on undergarments, buttoning your shirt, buttoning your pants, pulling up the zipper, and down to tying your shoes, these actions are made more difficult by hypotonia (low tone).

All of the therapies assist with achieving confidence and independence in these daily activities from the occupational therapist helping with buttons, zippers, and snaps; the physical therapist for the balance and lifting of extremities, and finally we cannot forget the speech therapist when all else fails and they need to ask or sign for help. This is an integral part of development to have an abundance of patience as they try, try again, fail, try again until finally they master the skill. Remember FAIL stands for "First Attempt In Learning."

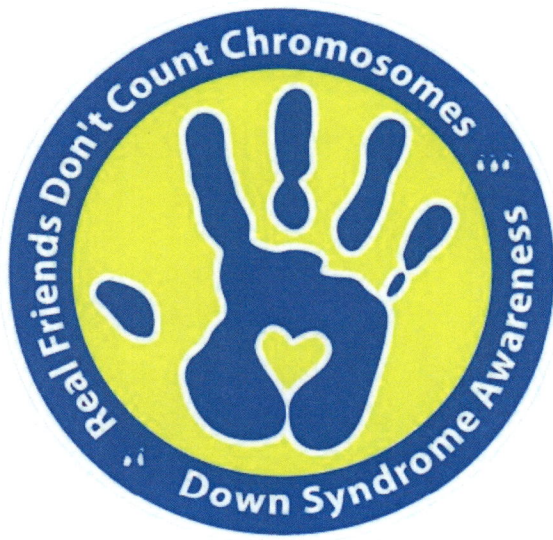

God doesn't give special
kids to special parents.
He takes ordinary,
imperfect people, and
gifts them with his
greatest treasures.
And therein, he creates
special parents.

Day 16

I'm Old Enough Now

Logan has always LOVED Halloween! He has usually dressed up as a super hero/movie/cartoon character. This year for the first time EVER, he announced he will not dress to trick or treat and instead hand out candy. He told me he is old enough.

I wrote before how we celebrate each milestone/accomplishment no matter how small. He is almost nineteen. I agreed with him and smiled, happy he came to this conclusion on his own and a little sad we are not trick or treating after nineteen plus years with him and his sister.

When kids come to your door for Halloween, remember a few things.

- They may not be able to verbalize trick or treat or thank you for the candy, they may be non verbal, hearing impaired, or may have another challenge that may be perceived as rude on the receiving end.
- They may not really be dressed in what we consider "Halloween" attire due to sensory issues. Even if they don't have a need of some kind, at my house, there is no age limit, everyone gets candy.
- Be empathic. It's a fun night for most but a little stressful and overwhelming for others.

Friends don't let friend's count chromosomes ❤

Day 17

"That Mother..."

I am not special; I married my high school sweetheart, have two children, a girl and a boy, and just try to navigate this crazy life, it's really that simple. Somewhere along the way, I turned into "that mom."

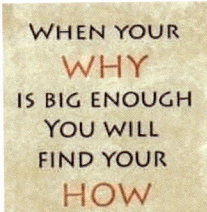

WHEN YOUR WHY IS BIG ENOUGH YOU WILL FIND YOUR HOW

The mom who honestly thinks her child with Down syndrome would be an asset rather than a liability, as an employee to your company.

Who thinks her son doesn't have to "keep up" to be included, social, accepted, and make a difference.

The mom who cares when you use the word "retarded," even when they argue that they "didn't mean your son." And the list goes on.

I'm that mom for both my daughter and my son, but I am not special. Any mom lucky enough to have children becomes "that mom." My daughter, a mother figure from almost the beginning, a protector of her brother, moves closer and closer toward being "that sister," which in turn will prepare her to be "that mom" if she chooses that path.

If I don't advocate for my children, who will? If I don't role model an advocate, how will they learn to self-advocate? Being an advocate can be for something minor like what clothes they want to wear, or on a larger scale, where they want to go to school or hold a job.

Friends don't let friend's count chromosomes ♥

#friendsdon'tletfriendscountchromosomes #specialneedsmom #downsyndrome #downsyndromeawareness #proudmom #selfadvocate #personfirstlanguage #therock #dwaynjohnson #markwahlberg #normalisboring #diversity

Day 18

Socialites

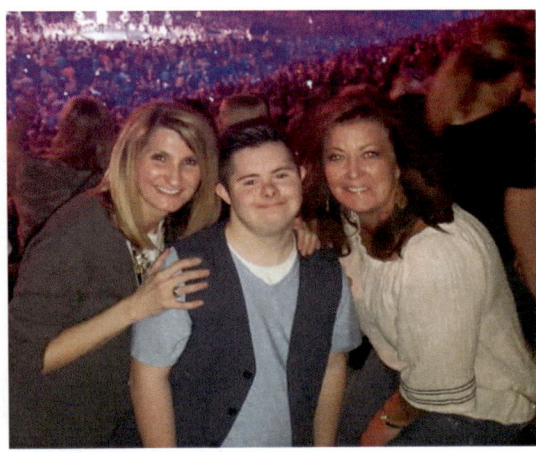

"More alike than different" is a topic I spoke on many times when Logan was in elementary school and one I post about every year. I spotlighted his favorite things, so the other kids could realize just how much alike we all are.

Now that Logan is a teenager, it's an even more important point, instead of staring or avoiding, start a conversation.

Logan loves to talk on certain topics. He will tell you he LOVES music, eating out, movies, hanging with friends, watching the Eagles game, basketball, going to concerts, and just being noticed and included. He has seen many concerts, Maroon 5, Nick Jonas, Justine Timberlake, Pink, Bruno Mars, and most recently Shawn Mendes.

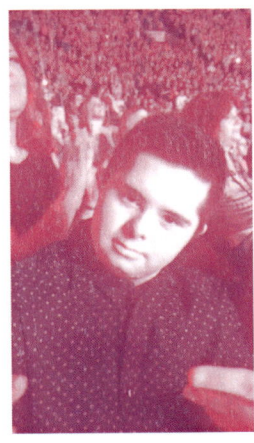

Sometimes when I take him to concerts, I may hardly know any songs, but his enthusiasm and passion for music makes it always a great time!

The Passion They Chose

We cannot pick or choose our children's passions, we can only support them. Some kids may not like sports, some may excel at sports, and some may like sports but have no coordination just like the inclusion.

The same goes for any "LIKE" we have in life. The things we are passionate about are not learned and cannot be changed, just nourished. ALL your children need is support, no matter their ability, your support in their interests, their passions, the little things that make them individuals and their personalities shine.

Whether they like to read, sing, kick or hit a ball, be their biggest cheerleader. I have found over the years Logan has so much enthusiasm for the things he loves, it transfers to me. I never really watched a basketball game before Logan professed his love for the sport, now I have even taken him to see the Sixer's and totally enjoyed it. Who knew?

Friends don't let friend's count chromosomes ❤

#therock #dwaynjohnson #markwahlberg #normalisboring #diversity

Day 19

Sexuality and Abuse

"Me too"…more recently this movement has swallowed our culture, although building respect for those who deserve much, much more, missing the target on sexual assault and harassment that does not discriminate.

A study found that children with intellectual disability were four times more likely to be sexually abused (Sullivan & Knutson, 2000).

Women are sexually assaulted more often when compared to men, whether they have a disability or not, so men with disabilities are often over-looked.

Researchers have found men with disabilities are twice as likely to become a victim of sexual violence compared to men without disabilities (The Roeher Institute, 1995). Also, abuse is typically more severe and more likely to occur multiple times and is more likely to be repeated for a longer period of time.

Imagine being socially or intellectually inept and unable to recount or report these unwanted advances or situations. Logan cannot answer simple questions most days, even what he did earlier in his day, unless the question is specific, let alone telling a situation that happened he may or may not know was wrong and caused him to feel uncomfortable. The "wh" questions are the most difficult for him, who, what, when, where, and why. We may never know.

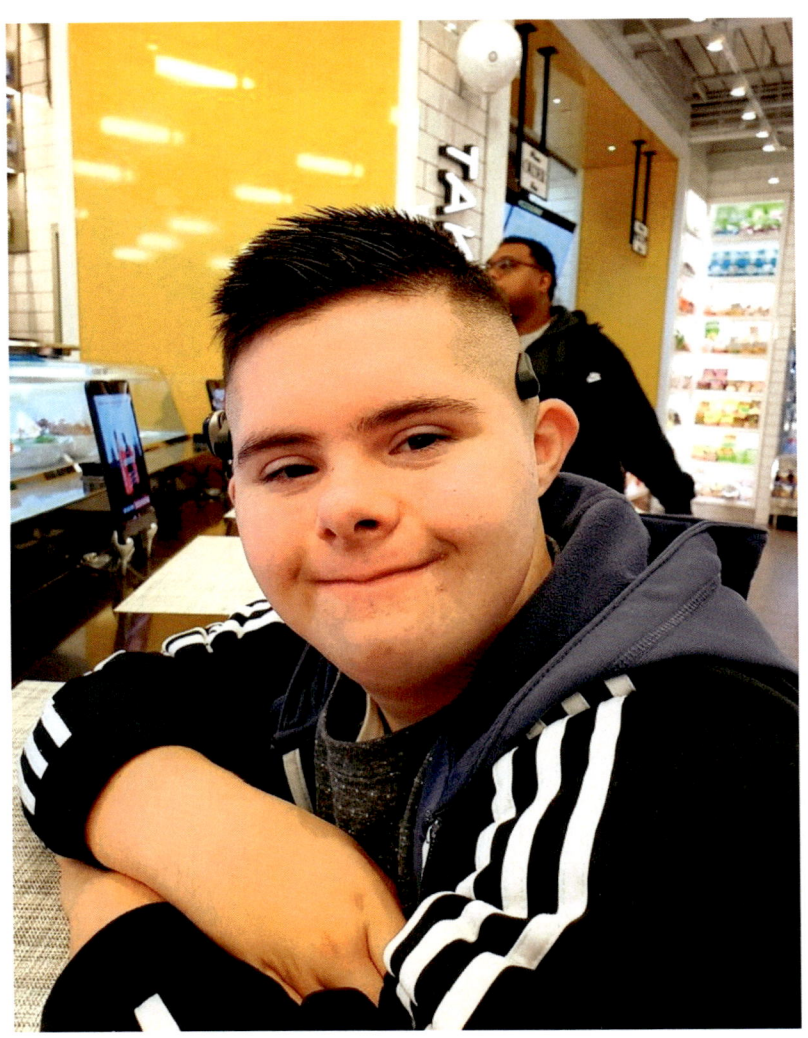

Day 20

The Down Syndrome Mind

People with Down syndrome are born with an extra copy of chromosome 21, which carries the APP gene. By age forty, almost all people with Down syndrome have these plaques from the extra APP, along with other protein deposits, which cause problems with how brain cells function. Estimates suggest fifty percent or more of people with Down syndrome will develop dementia due to Alzheimer's disease as they age. People with Down syndrome begin to show symptoms of Alzheimer's disease in their fifties or sixties (https://www.nia.nih.gov/… /alzheimers-disease-people-down-sy…).

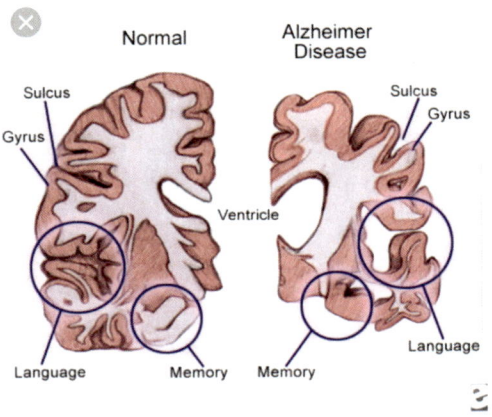

The life expectenancy of an individual with Down syndrome has gone from twenty-five in 1983 to an average of sixty years of age. Mostly due to the fact the children with Down syndrome are not routinely institutionalized after birth. I could not imagine not having Logan as part of our household. He definitely completes us.

Day 21

Different in the Best Way

Talk to your children about DIVERSITY.

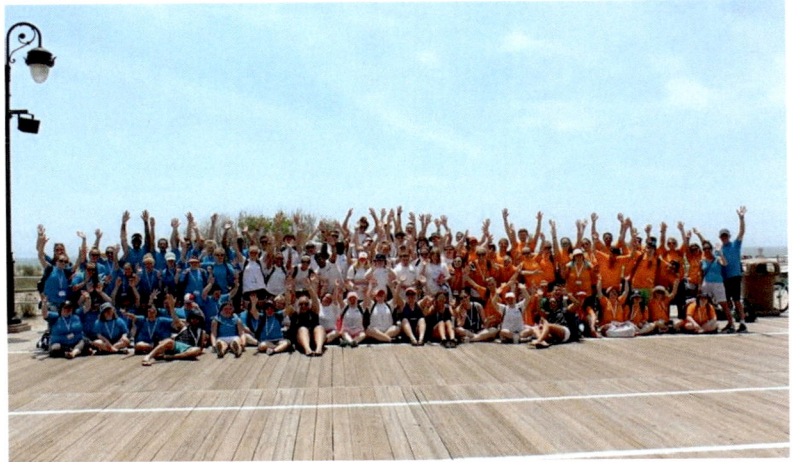

Some people have brown hair, some blonde, some eat through a tube, some wear hearing aids, some have wheelchairs, some have a tank with a tube in their nose to help them breathe, and some have Down syndrome.

Let your child ask questions, especially to Logan and me. I cannot tell you how many children and adults just stand there and stare. It makes for an uncomfortable moment to say the least.

So please talk to your children. Diversity is a beautiful thing, whether it's your ethnicity or a disability, no matter your height or ability level. The world would be tedious, dull, monotonous, repetitive, just plain boring place without diversity.

Have a question? Please ask me!

Diversity

Diversity, we hear this word often throughout our daily life. Do we really understand the power of this word's meaning? Diversity simply put means each individual is unique. To a special needs parent, this simple definition defines us. No one understands this better than a household where "normal" is in the eye of the beholder and everyday may be a new "normal."

Understanding diversity, it's a broad subject really, encompassing gender, social-economic status, race, ability level, and religious beliefs. Being diverse is natural really! We are diverse because we are all different with the exception of identical twins, and even then, having the same DNA, they can have different personalities, beliefs, and friends. Being diverse really is just being. Our definition of normal is changed by every individual's perception and diversity.

Friends don't let friend's count chromosomes ❤

#personfirstlanguage #therock #dwaynjohnson #markwahlberg #normalisboring #diversity

Day 22

Milestones

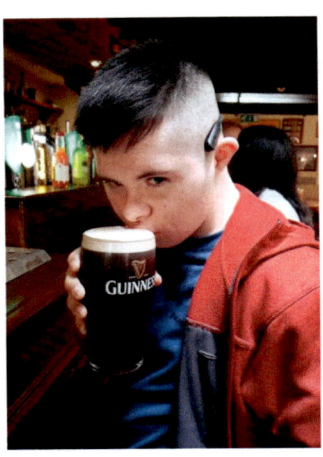

Children and adults with Down syndrome hit their milestones just like their typical peers but in their own time.

Due to low tone and other challenges, children and adults with Down syndrome will experience delays. Since Logan did and still does experience delays in development, physically, mentally and cognitively, we celebrate EVERY milestone, no matter how small.

I have NEVER had faith in Down syndrome charts or expected behavior data. I've told the school more than once when they pull out their charts, my son is NOT data.

We are still celebrating age appropriate behavior. He asked and attended prom with his girlfriend again this year. In Ireland, just like any other teen, Logan could not wait to drink a Guinness and try Jameson. Earlier this year, he walked at graduation, had a big party, and loves to drink his coffee every morning just like everyone else. Logan lives life with his whole being enjoying EVERY minute.

Friends don't let friend's count chromosomes ♥

Consider this

We were never stuck on Logan making his milestones. I am not sure why, maybe because he was second born and we had a twenty-three-month-old running around the house, too? I'm not saying we didn't take every therapy offered and do ALL the exercises they recommended. I just felt like it would come when he was ready. Or not, but either way, my worrying and stressing would not change it.

I remember when Logan was about ten-months-old and we were literally teaching him to crawl. We would have him on all fours and move his legs in a crawling motion, so his brain and muscles would eventually do it on their own from muscle memory. Guess what, Logan never crawled, maybe scooted but never crawled. After months and months of therapies and both of us repeating the therapist's routines with very little progress. Then one day, Logan pulled himself up on the edge of the sofa and walked. The funny thing was I was so frustrated, and just when I had finally reached accepting this was not going to happen, there he went off, walking around the house. It didn't matter that he didn't crawl or reach that milestone. There have been other experiences through the years that mirror this one, and almost EVERY time, just when I have reached the mindset of "OK, this is OK, he may never do (this)," I am happy to say he proves me wrong.

Day 23

Nothing Stops Sports

Logan was diagnosed with Atlanto Axial Instability at an extremely young age, which is an inoperable condition of his spine at the base of his neck.

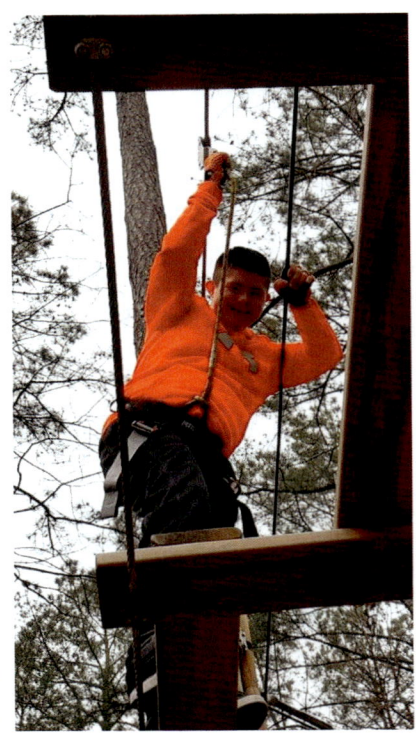

Atlantoaxial instability (AAI) affects 10–20% of individuals with Down syndrome (DS). The condition is mostly asymptomatic and diagnosed on radiography by an enlarged anterior atlanto-odon'toid distance. (Cervical spine abnormalities associated with Down syndrome - NCBI) Luckily for Logan, his diagnosis did not carry limitations for him with any aspect of his daily life. After fifteen years at an orthopedic who specializes in this diagnosis, he was discharged from his care two months ago in the fall of 2019. Although Logan is "vertically challenged," his favorite sport is basketball.

Consider this

When Logan was diagnosed with AAI, I thought wow, this is it, no more sports, no more roller coasters, no more of most of his favorite activities. We were getting ready to leave for Disney in the coming weeks, and my first

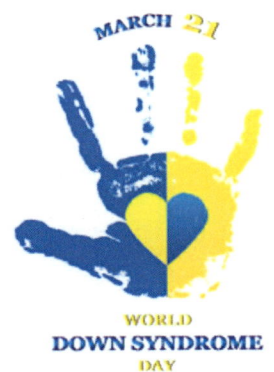

thought was how are we going to go to Disney World and not ride a roller coaster. My mind was racing in all directions, like how am I going to help him get exercise and stay active to help with his weight, how can I help him stay healthy? I am an active person and thrive on being active together, and when this diagnosis was confirmed, I thought, well, that's the end of that. Then I stopped, took a breath, and thought how many diagnosis have we had since Logan was born? We have taken each one on stride, not to say we didn't have a moment of processing the emotions attached to the words, but honestly we have a pretty good track record for getting through each and every day, not to brag but so far its 100%.

Friends don't let friend's count chromosomes ♥

#friendsdon'tletfriendscountchromosomes #specialneedsmom #downsyndrome #downsyndromeawareness #proudmom #selfadvocate #personfirstlanguage #therock #dwaynjohnson #markwahlberg #normalisboring

Day 24

Sticks and Stones

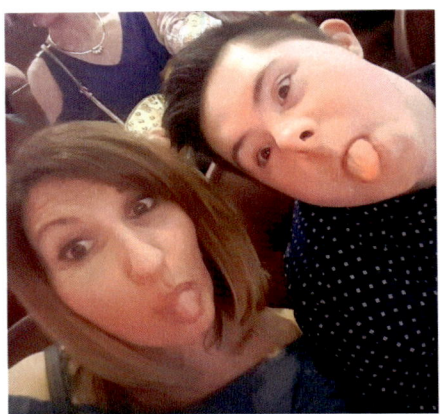

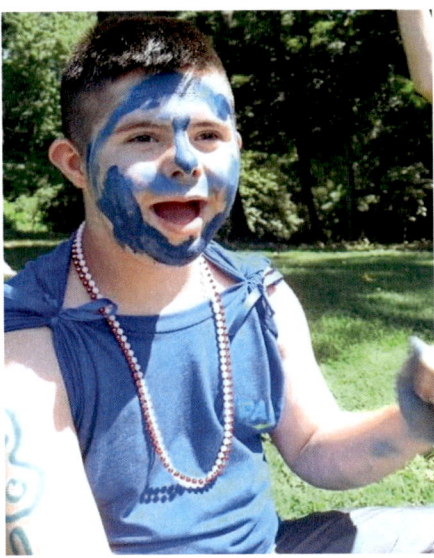

When I was growing up, we used to say, "Sticks and stones can break my bones, but names can never hurt me." But we all know that is not true. Words can be hurtful, and once spoken, cannot be taken back. The word "normal" by definition, [Adj. conforming to a standard; usual, typical, or expected, noun - the usual, average, or typical state or condition].

I am proud to say my household is NOT normal, sometimes close to ab-normal in a whole different definition. Even before Logan. I can assure you what I consider a "normal" day in my house is not what a "normal day" looks like in your house. I am proud of both of my children for not being normal. Normal is boring. Down-right normal.

Consider this

Normal, it is a common enough word, meaning usual, typical, and if you ask me, down-right boring. Who wants to be normal? I thought I did growing up, I wanted to be like everyone else, not draw attention to myself and blend in. WHAT WAS I THINKING! We get one chance at making memories in this crazy life, and let's not make them normal. Let's make them exciting, happy, loud, attention drawing, do what makes you happy moments in time.

Friends don't let friend's count chromosomes ♥

#friendsdon'tletfriendscountchromosomes #specialneedsmom #downsyndro me #downsyndromeawareness #proudmom #selfadvocate #personfirstlangua ge #therock #dwaynjohnson #markwahlberg #normalisboring

Day 25

Finding the Path Forward

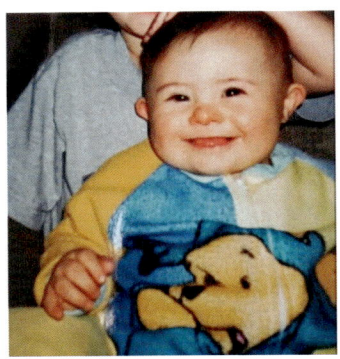

As an adult with Down syndrome, Logan still has a range of needs, abilities, and desires, just like any other group of people. Adults with DS have different experiences; some will learn to drive, have relationships, and live almost entirely on their own. With our support, Logan will have a rich, fulfilling life and feel part of his community, and whatever that looks like for him is OK with us.

Educating ourselves on all the different departments that will benefit Logan as he graduates and enters into adulthood: OVR, MHIDD, Medicaid, Social Security, guardianship vs power of attorney, etcetera, is a full-time job and at times feels like it requires an additional degree.

I am not sure if I am doing it right, but I do know I am doing what I believe is best for his future.

Friends don't let friend's count chromosomes ♥

Day 26

Patients Pays Dividends

There was an EMG study that showed the average person uses 72.52 microvolts of energy to initiate voice production, but individuals with Down syndrome need to use 131.57 microvolts; it takes almost twice as much effort for a person living with Down syndrome to obtain the same result as it does for us {https://library.down-syndrome.org/.../voice-people-down-synd.../).

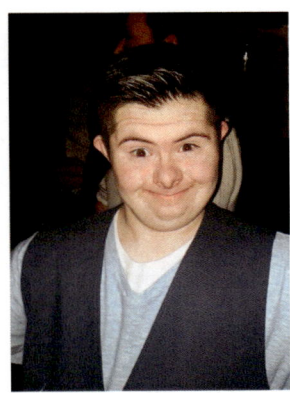

So what does this mean...

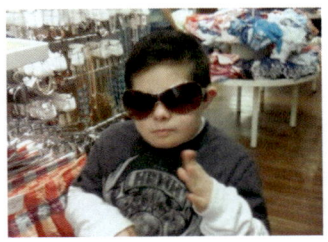

It took Logan longer than his typical peers to speak. To prevent Logan from becoming frustrated, we taught ourselves and him sign language, so he could relay to us what he wanted/needed. As Logan has gotten older, he developed a stutter from his brain working faster than his mouth muscles can interpret and get it out.

When conversing with a person living with DS, remember, be patient, allow the individual to process what is being said, and give ample time to answer. Don't answer for them.

Friends don't let friend's count chromosomes ♥

#friendsdon'tletfriendscountchromosomes #specialneedsmom #downsyndrome #downsyndromeawareness

Day 27

Down Syndrome Awareness Month

"It is time for parents to teach young people early on, in diversity there is beauty and there is strength." Maya Angelou

ACCEPTANCE; we all want to be accepted in one way or another. As a parent of Logan, ACCEPTANCE is what I have thought of often throughout his life. In the beginning, it was my acceptance of his diagnosis, his limitations, my expectations, and how I "thought" life should be. As the years pass, it has shifted to society, and their acceptance of my truly amazingly funny thoughtful empathetic man, who if you don't take the time to get to know, YOU are truly the one missing out.

Friends don't let friend's count chromosomes ❤

#friendsdon'tletfriendscountchromosomes #specialneedsmom #downsyndrome #downsyndromeawareness #proudmom #selfadvocate #acceptance #therock

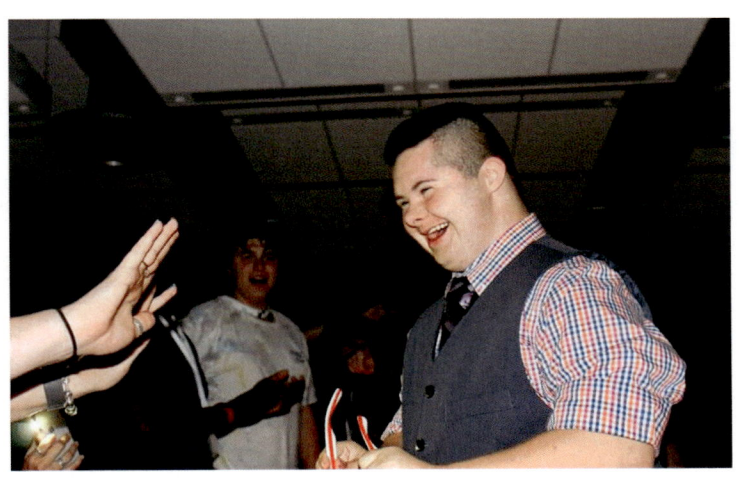

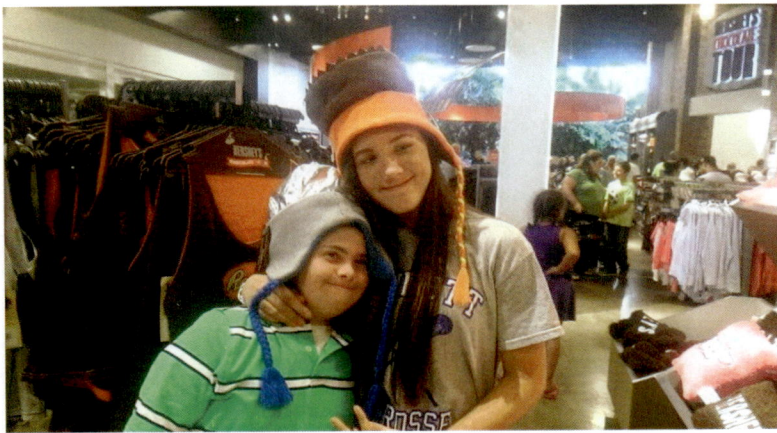

Day 28

Communication

People, first, language is simple…

All you need to do is put the person's names or "girl," "kid," "baby" before the words "Down syndrome." Just say, "Child with Down syndrome" instead of "Down syndrome child." Down syndrome does not define my child; it's just a small part of him. Logan is not Down syndrome.

Friends don't let friend's count chromosomes ❤

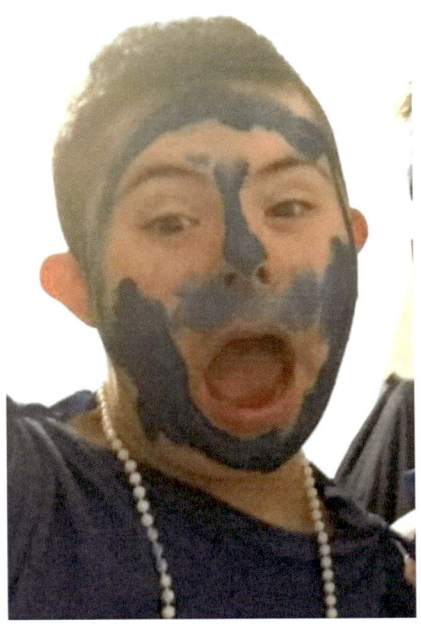

Day 29

Select Learning

We are all constantly transitioning through our lives from grade to grade, job to job. The period following high school is full of excitement but can present many challenges.

Finding programs for young adults with special needs is challenging.

The selections of programs that are available are depressingly minimal. As our young adults age, our choices for programming decrease in comparison to transition process for our typical young adults.

If you own a business, hire me. If you don't have adults with needs working or volunteering at your place of employment, ask why not? If you are employed by a college and don't have a life skills college program....why not?

"Let's make the ceiling our new floor."

Friends don't let friend's count chromosomes 🖤

#friendsdon'tletfriendscountchromosomes #specialneedsmom #downsyndrome #downsyndromeawareness #proudmom #selfadvocate

Day 30

Down Syndrome Stats

Down syndrome continues to be an all too common chromosomal disorder. One in every 700 babies born in 2008 had Down syndrome (cdc.gov). Approximately one out of every 1,200 people (children, teens, and adults) living in the United States have Down syndrome.

Older mothers are more likely to have a baby affected by Down syndrome than younger mothers. The prevalence of Down syndrome increases as you age, most children with Down syndrome are statistically born to younger mothers only because the younger age group is giving birth to more babies than older age groups. I was twenty-nine when I had Logan with no risk factors.

Friends don't let friend's count chromosomes ♥

#friendsdon'tletfriendscountchromosomes #specialneedsmom #downsyndrome #downsyndromeawareness #proudmom #selfadvocate

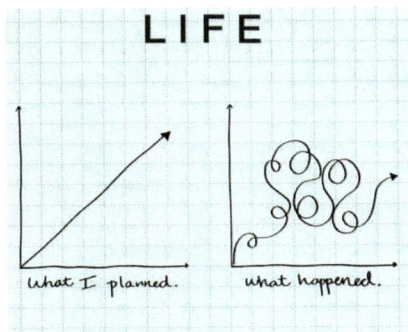

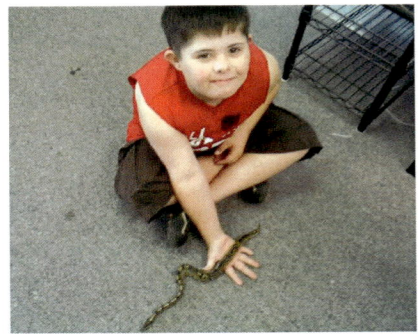

Day 31

What May Seem Different, is Still the Same

31 things to remember about Logan:

1. Started to walk at the age of three
2. Still has baby teeth at age nineteen
3. LOVES and MISSES his sister every day she's away
4. Has had thirteen surgeries, ALL WITH A SMILE
5. People first language; Logan is not Down syndrome
6. Never complains, no matter how sick he might get
7. He wants you to stop using the "R" word, in all context
8. He has the same wants and needs as you
9. He feels "ALL" feelings and emotions
10. Wants to be treated with respect
11. Understands much more than most give him credit for.
12. LOVES movies and music
13. Sees multiple specialists, has numerous appointments and still smiles everyday
14. Most empathetic person you will ever meet, regardless of social status, gender, age, ability level, ethnicity, color, religion or political affiliation
15. Wants to live in Ireland with his Dad
16. Can dead-lift 195 pounds!
17. Has the best sarcastic sense of humor...and doesn't know it!
18. When he smiles, his eyes reflect his heart
19. Can throw a fierce ax
20. Best Altar Server ever, with his buddy Deacon Madonna

21. Went zip lining and had a blast
22. The Philadelphia 76ers is Logan's favorite team and Mike Scott his favorite player
23. Logan is the definition of unconditional love and gives the best HUGS!
24. Logan has a memory like an elephant
25. Exhibits the spirit of Christmas everyday
26. Logan doesn't "suffer" from Down Syndrome, nor is he defined by societies definitions
27. Has the best aunts and uncles ever! (His words)
28. Pee-Pop is his best friend
29. He asks, "How's Grammy" EVERY DAY!
30. LOVES, HUGS, and SNUGGLES MOMMY EVERY MORNING
31. He sees the good in everyone; the world would be a better place if we were more like Logan

Just the Beginning

And so we come to the end of our thirty-one days. Don't fool yourself…it's only the beginning. I know it may not seem like it at times; if you are reading as lucky new parents, but as I suggested when we started our journey… BREATHE…and now I want to suggest you add…SMILE! Everyday won't be easy or good, but there will be good in everyday.

Your heart grows ten-fold, your soul becomes one with your new family member, your family and friends huddle around you and pick you up when you feel down, but most importantly, you and your significant other have a new BEST FRIEND who no matter your day, no matter your mood, will lift you up by just coming into the room.

It's twenty years for us now, and I can assure you, we have yet to see a special family that is not incredibly happy and always lives in the mindset of NO REGRETS. In fact the level of fulfillment you will experience becomes overwhelming, an altruistic life experience, as your new family grows into their life…together!

Don't change your goals "because this is different"…enhance your goals because this makes the difference. Nothing should change. You have a new partner in your goals who will make reaching those goals even sweeter. ANYTHING is possible, and it begins with YOU!

Friends don't let friend's count chromosomes ❤

Special Thanks

Kayla

Grammy

Me-Mom

Pee-Pop

Pop-Pop

All my Aunts and Uncles

Aunt Maggie

Denise Marino

Miss Helen

Glasgow (Bev)

Ms. Danese (Judy)

Connolly (Joanne)

Stampone (Nicole)

Dr. Karsch

Ryan McKeon

"SHARON!" McQuaide

"Dude" McQuaide (Jim)

"Friend" Shelly Azen

Nadya & Ed

Dr. Parks

Kennet HS Basketball

Dr. Godovin

Dr. Monica Lepore (and students)

Mr. Lentz

Dylan Badger

Kyle

Camp BourneLyf Team
Camp Pals Team
Special Olympics Team
Deacon Jim Madonna

"It takes a village," and we are blessed each and every one of you have brought something special to Logan's life. Our "village" is truly blessed because you are part of it.